ICD-10 is an international medical code system that describes roughly 76,000 diseases, symptoms, abnormal findings, and external causes of injury. The 10th edition was published in 1992 by the World Health Organization. The United States is transitioning to this standard by October 1, 2014. ICD-11 is expected to be published in 2015.

This book is a collaboration among artists representing a diverse background in healthcare across the United States.

Welcome to the initial encounter edition.

Enjoy,
Niko

R14.1

Gas pain

Kendra Zueck – Mixed Media
Kendra studied Art and Design at the University of Wisconsin - Eau Claire. She enjoys Madison today for the tastier things in life: music, art, and craft beer.

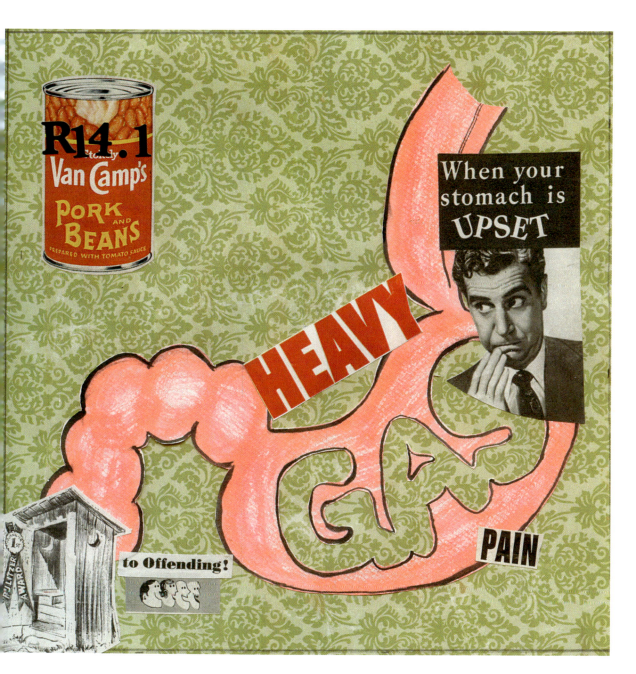

R46.1

Bizarre personal appearance

Chelsea Wittenbaugh – Watercolor on Canvas 11" x 15"
Chelsea is an artist, maybe a painter, a poet, a glue aficionado, and most definitely an existentialist. She currently lives a glitter-filled, hippie-punk, fantastically colorful life while working for a healthcare IT company in Denver, CO.

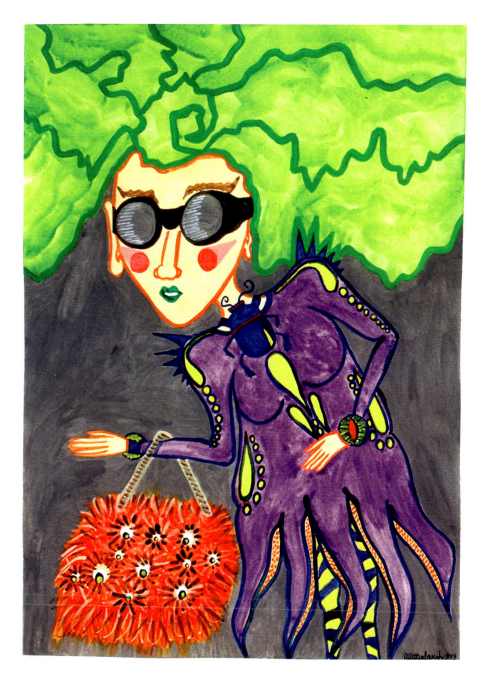

T50.5x6A

Underdosing of appetite depressants, initial encounter

Sara Albrecht-Chubrilo – Ink on Paper 8"x10"
Sara works at Nordic, the largest Epic-only consulting firm in the country. She has a love for doodling, laughter, and the ridiculous.

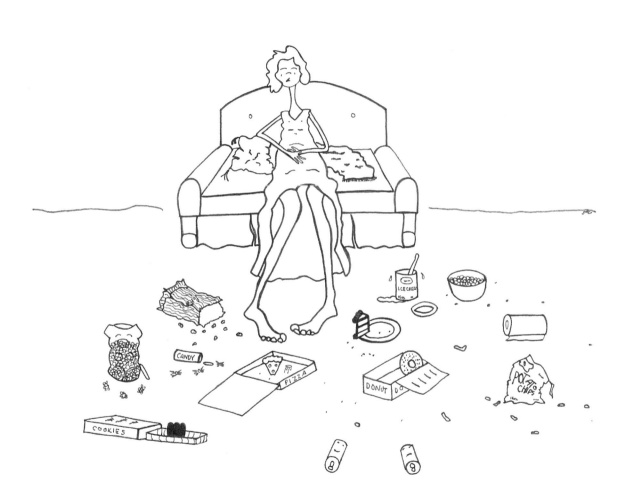

T63.442S

Toxic effect of venom of bees, intentional self-harm, sequela

Jon Lyons – Pen and Ink Wash on Paper 8"x10"
Jon Lyons is an artist, illustrator, cartoonist/animator, designer, and stand up comedian living in Chicago.

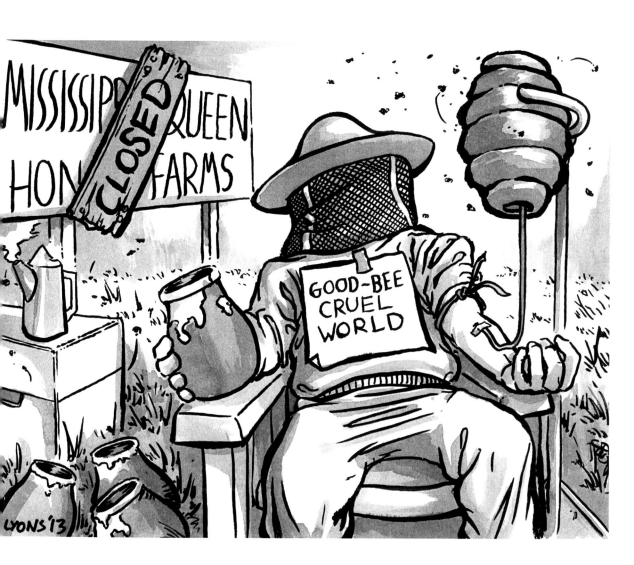

T78.04xA

Anaphylactic shock due to fruits and vegetables, initial encounter

Jimmy Xu – Finger on iPad
Jimmy is a medical student at the University of Wisconsin. He is looking forward to one day using this ICD-10 code.

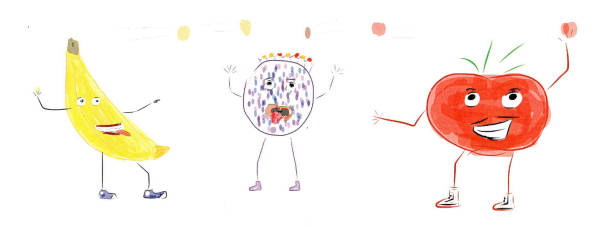

Little did they know that the young mast cell possessed an uncontrollable power.

V00.01xD

Pedestrian on foot injured in collision with roller-skater, subsequent encounter

James Lloyd – Digital
James is the co-founder of 100health and is a wizard with EMR integration. He worked at Epic for six years in various roles including technical services, EDI, and software development. Needless to say, he's a productivity mastermind. In fact, he outsourced his art for this book.

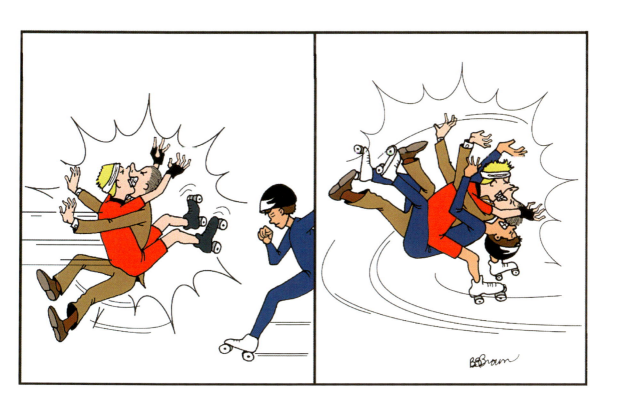

V32.1xxS

Passenger in three-wheeled motor vehicle injured in collision with two- or three-wheeled motor vehicle in nontraffic accident, sequela

Katie Vice – Photography, Digital Media
Katie has been working in Quality Assurance at Epic since 2010.
She has been making art for as long as she can remember.

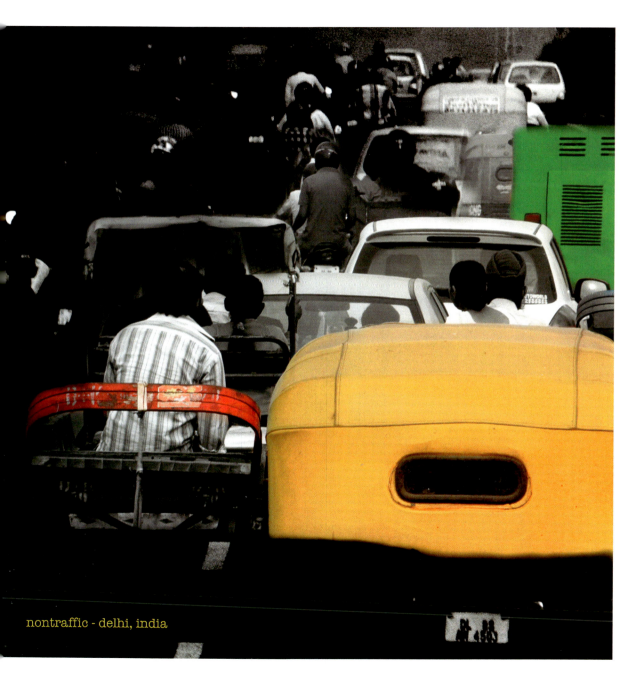

V61.6xxD

Passenger in heavy transport vehicle injured in collision with pedal cycle in traffic accident, subsequent encounter

Sarah Sandock– Pencil on Paper, Digital Color 8" x 8"
Sarah is a biomedical engineer who ventured into healthcare by founding Dock Technologies in Madison, WI.

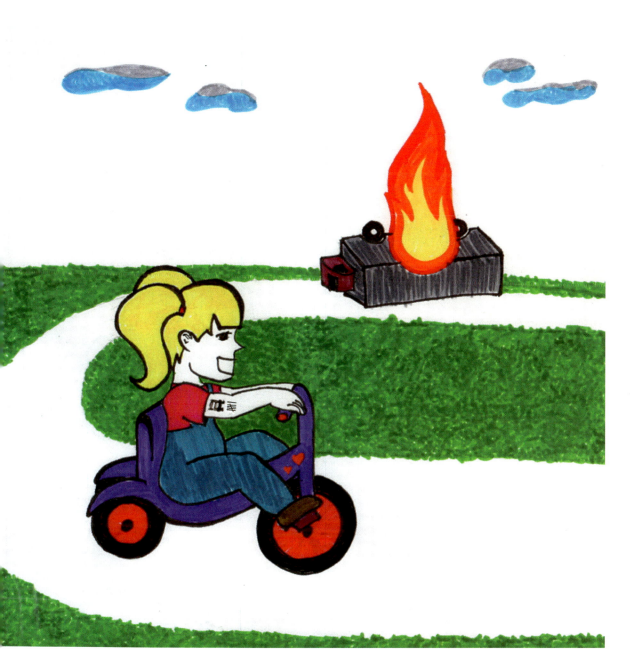

V91.07xD

Burn due to water-skis on fire, subsequent encounter

Sarah Bottjen – Acrylic and Nail Polish on Canvas 12" x 9"
Sarah is currently an Epic project manager on the emergency department team. In her free time, she like to paint with acrylics on found objects. Her largest works are showcased on Epic's campus, where 8 walls exhibit her cave art. She's a French, Chinese and Arabic language fanatic, with a potential interest in emergency medicine in the future.

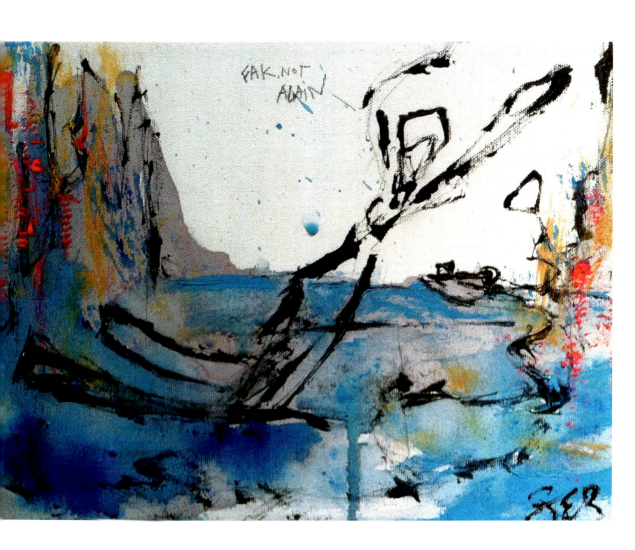

V91.30xA

Hit or struck by falling object due to accident on merchant ship, initial encounter

James Lloyd – Digital
James is the co-founder of 100health and is a wizard with EMR integration. He worked at Epic for six years in various roles including technical services, EDI, and software development. Needless to say, he's a productivity mastermind. In fact, he outsourced his art for this book.

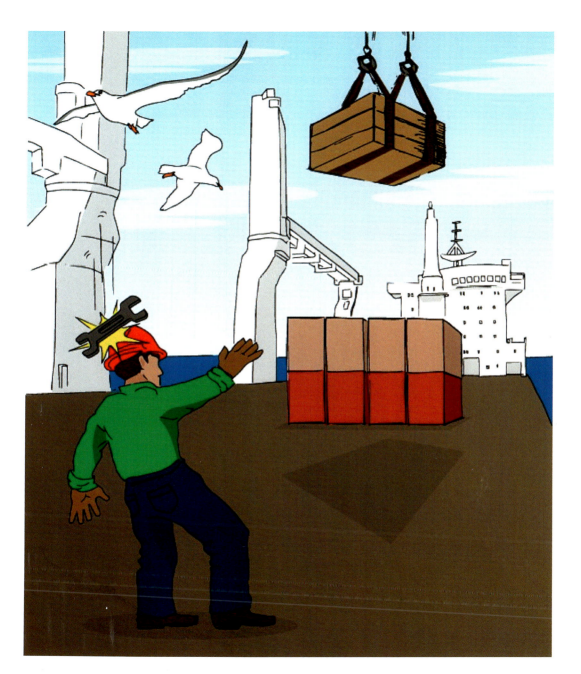

V93.54xD

Explosion on board sailboat, subsequent encounter

Beck Freidman – Finger on iPad
Beck is a technical services analyst at Epic, where he's known for his cave paintings in Epic's Deep Space auditorium. In his free time he enjoys all things automotive, rooting fanatically for Vanderbilt sports, and bowling with his team, the Golden Dragons.

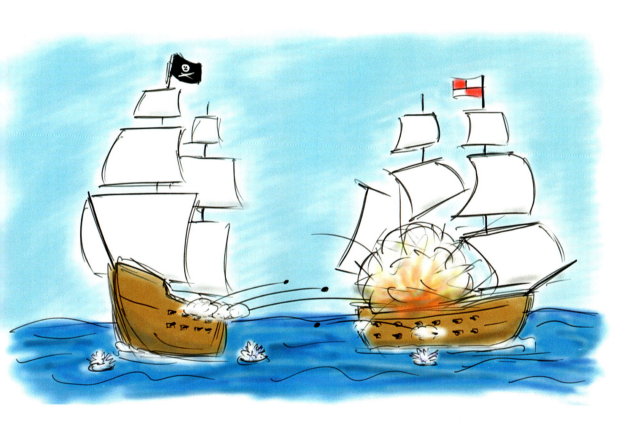

V95.42xA

Forced landing of spacecraft injuring occupant,
initial encounter

Sara Albrecht-Chubrilo – Ink on Paper 8"x10"
Sara works at Nordic, the largest Epic-only consulting firm in the country. She has a love for doodling, laughter, and the ridiculous.

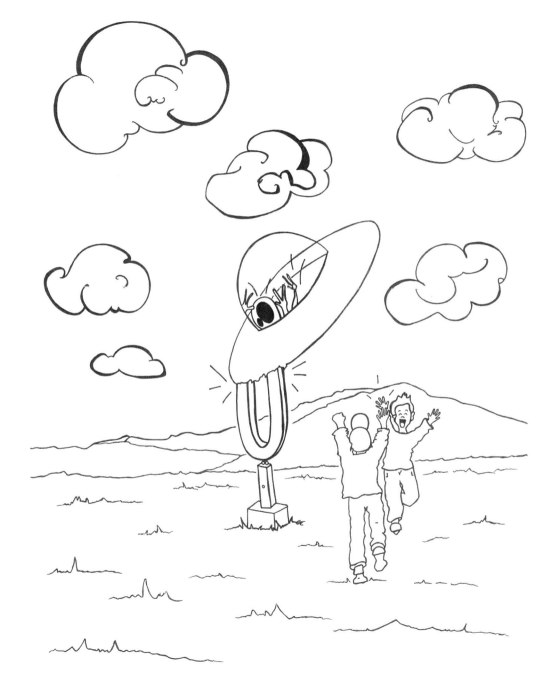

V96.00xS

Unspecified balloon accident injuring occupant, sequela

Erika Samlowski – Digital Media
Erika is a 2nd year medical student at the Medical College of Wisconsin.
She is interested in pursuing a career in reconstructive surgery.

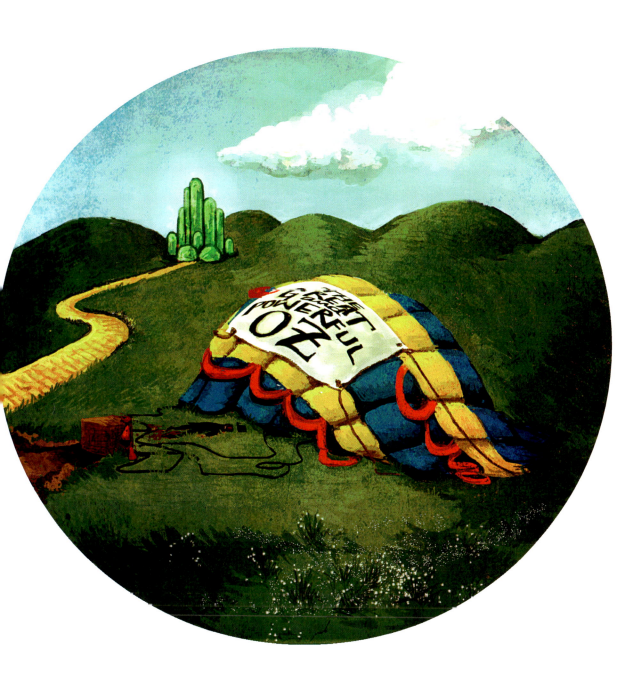

V97.33xD

Sucked into jet engine, subsequent encounter

Sarah Bottjen – Acrylic and Nailpolish on Canvas 10" x 13"
Sarah is currently an Epic project manager on the emergency department team. In her free time, she like to paint with acrylics on found objects. Her largest works are showcased on Epic's campus, where 8 walls exhibit her cave art. She's a French, Chinese and Arabic language fanatic, with a potential interest in emergency medicine in the future.

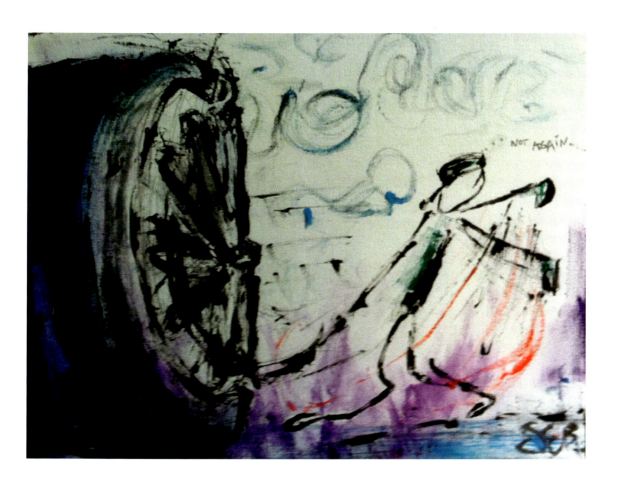

W01.190A

Fall on same level from slipping, tripping and stumbling with subsequent striking against furniture, initial encounter

James Lloyd – Digital
James is the co-founder of 100health and is a wizard with EMR integration. He worked at Epic for six years in various roles including technical services, EDI, and software development. Needless to say, he's a productivity mastermind. In fact, he outsourced his art for this book.

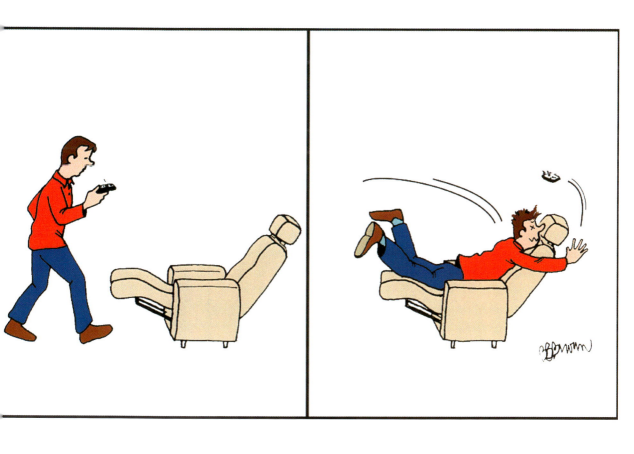

W04.xxxS
Fall while being carried or supported by other persons, sequela

W60.xxxA
Contact with nonvenemous plant thorns and spines and sharp leaves, initial encounter

Maggie Gosselar – 12" x 15" Markers on Paper
Maggie Gosselar (known in some circles as the Glock Ness Monster) is a unprofessional artist and roller derby girl from Madison, WI.

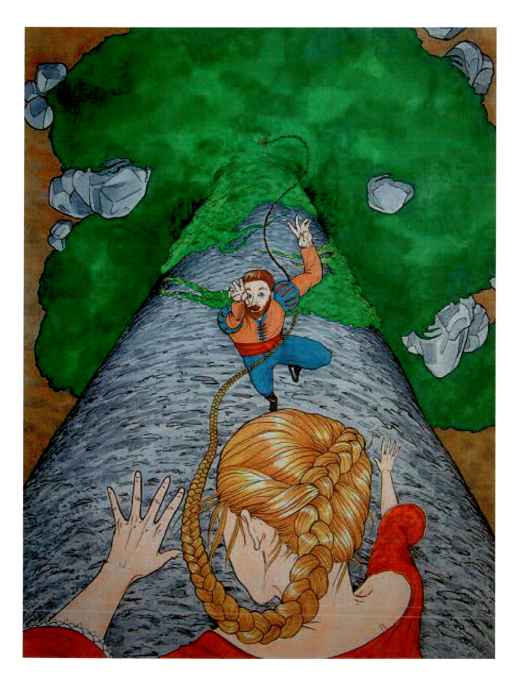

W21.00xA

Struck by hit or thrown ball,
unspecified type,
initial encounter

Kendra Zueck – Mixed Media
Kendra studied Art and Design at the University of Wisconsin - Eau Claire. She enjoys Madison today for the tastier things in life: music, art, and craft beer.

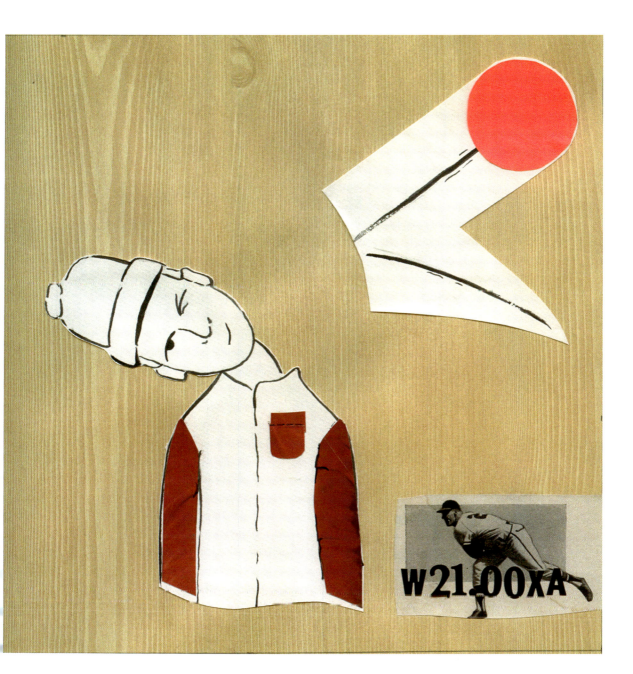

W56.21xS

Bitten by orca, sequela

Ellery Addington-White – Digital Media
Ellery is the Student Director at the Center For Entrepreneurship
and Liberal Education at Beloit College in Wisconsin.

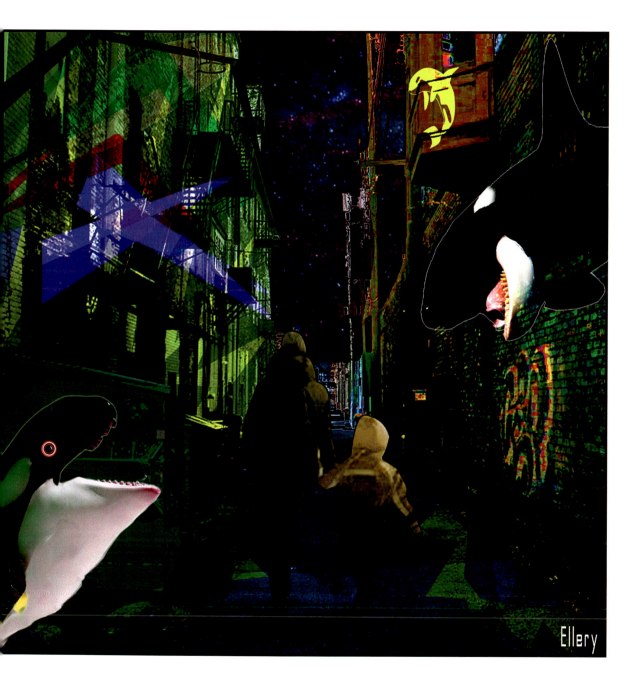

W56.22xA

Struck by orca, initial encounter

Ellery Addington-White – Digital Mixed Media
Ellery is the Student Director at the Center For Entrepreneurship and Liberal Education at Beloit College in Wisconsin.

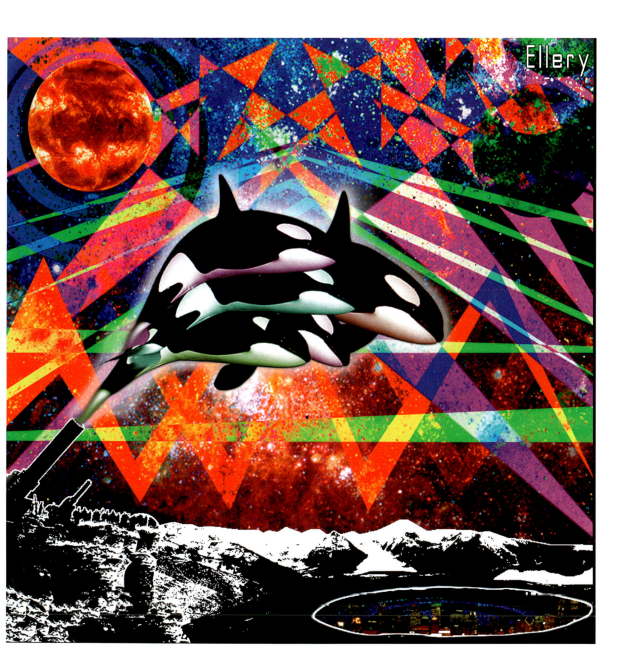

W56.22xD

Struck by orca, subsequent encounter

Alex Connelly – Digital Media
Alex is an artist from Madison, WI. His focus is in digital and analog/experimental photography as well as painting and mixed media.

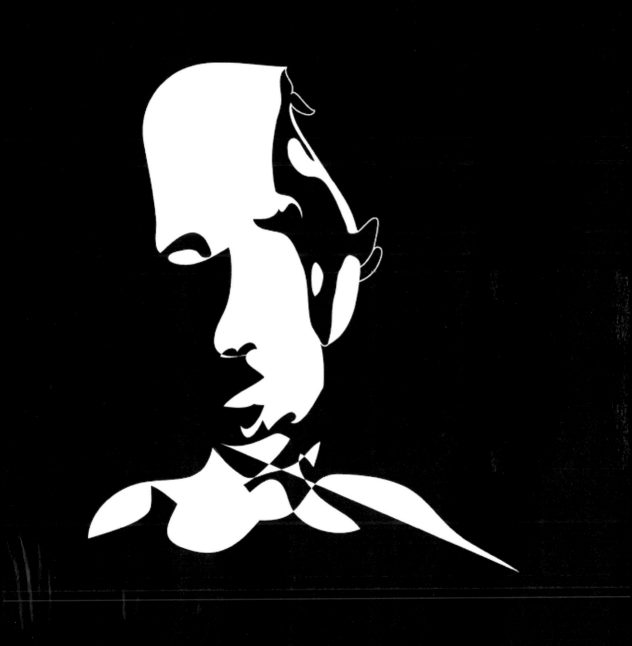

W56.49

Other contact with shark

Deb Berman – Oil on Canvas 60"x80"
Deb currently lives, paints, and eats donuts in the Brooklyn area.

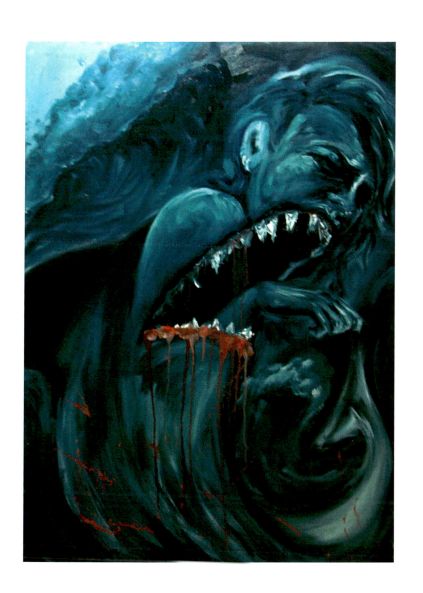

W59.02xA

Struck by a nonvenomous lizard, initial encounter

Katie Vice – Photography, Digital Media
Katie has been working in Quality Assurance at Epic since 2010.
She has a been making art for as long as she can remember.

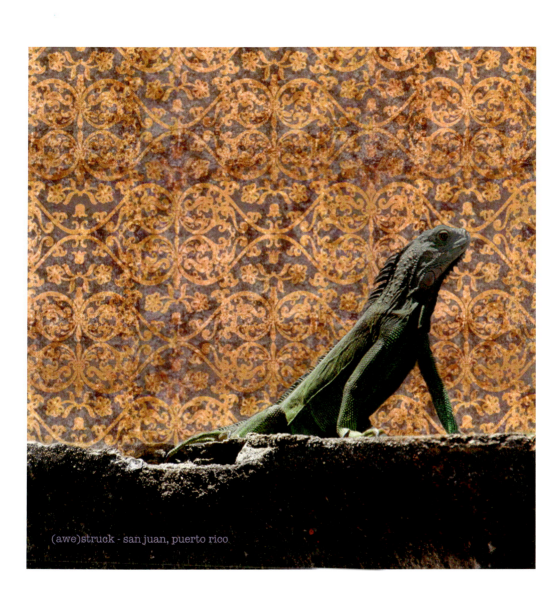
(awe)struck - san juan, puerto rico

W61.62
Struck by duck, sequela

Alex Connelly – Pen, Colored Pencil on Paper 10"x8"
Alex is an artist from Madison, WI. His focus is in digital and analog/experimental photography as well as painting and mixed media.

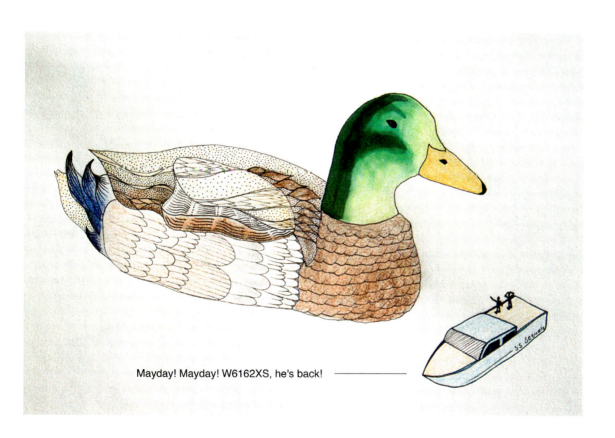
Mayday! Mayday! W6162XS, he's back!

X52

Prolonged stay in weightless environment

Jon Lyons – Digital Painting 8.5"x11"
Jon Lyons is an artist, illustrator, cartoonist/animator, designer, and stand up comedian living in Chicago.

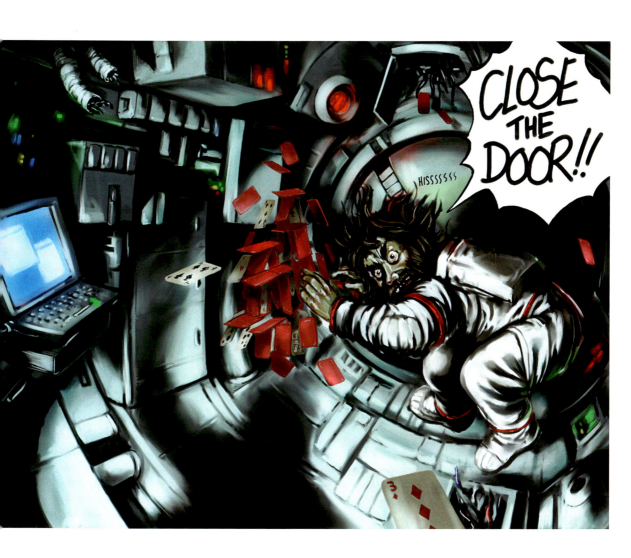

Y23.1

Hunting rifle discharge, undetermined intent

Kyle Pfister – Installation and Photograph
Kyle is the co-founder of public health innovation company Ninjas for Health. He's also an installation and performance artist whose current project "The Wisconsin Heritage Foundation" explores the intersection of beloved state traditions and the new wave of conservative politics.

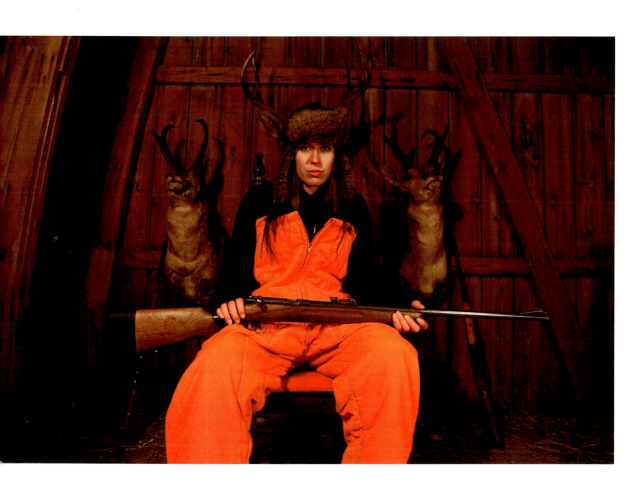

Y33

Other specified event, undetermined intent

Beck Freidman – Other Specified Media
Beck is an technical services analyst at Epic, where he's known for his cave paintings in Epic's Deep Space auditorium. In his free time he enjoys all things automotive, rooting fanatically for Vanderbilt sports, and bowling with his team, the Golden Dragons.

Y92.146

Swimming pool of prison as the place of occurrence of the external cause

Deb Berman – Acrylic, Gouache, Coffee on Canvas 18"x14"
Deb currently lives, paints, and eats donuts in the Brooklyn area.

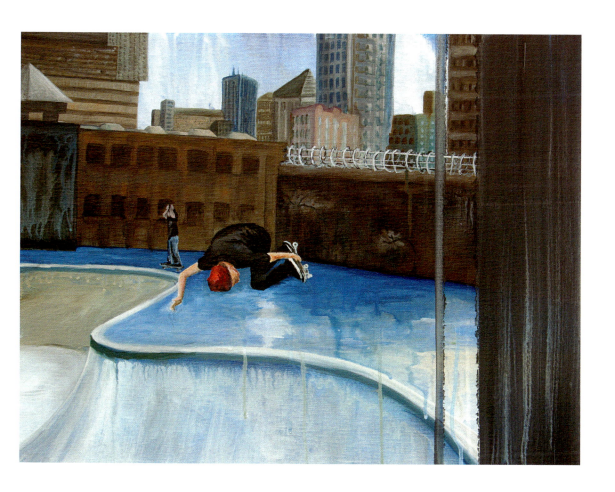

Y92.253

Opera house as the place of occurrence of the external cause

Laura Ash – Ink on Paper 8"x10"
Laura is a clinical herbalist, entrepreneur, and artist. She likes to laugh, play in the dirt, and laugh a lot.

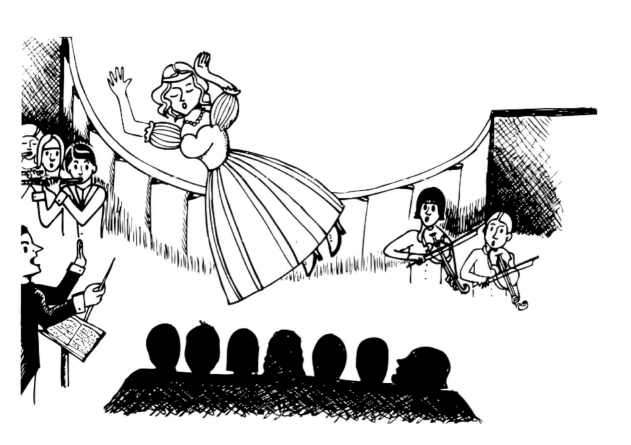

Y93.D1
Activity, knitting and crocheting

Alex Connelly – Photography
Alex iis an artist from Madison, WI. His focus is in digital and analog/experimental photography as well as painting and mixed media.

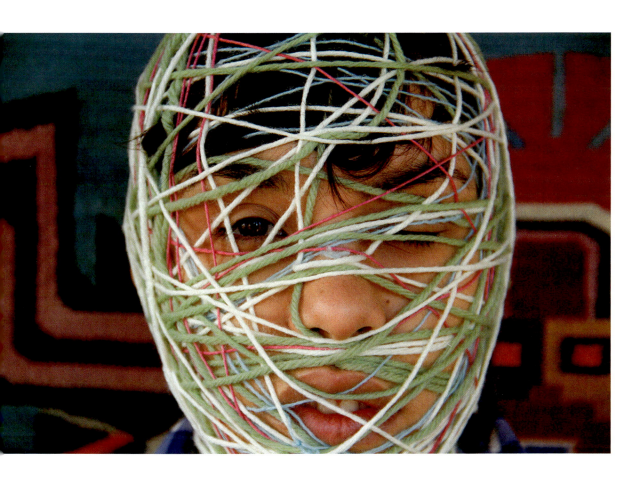

Y93.G2 Activity, grilling and smoking food

Y93.J1 Activity, piano playing

Phil Geiger - Digital Media
Phil is a project manager and blogger at Epic. He enjoys cycling and walking his dog and roommates.

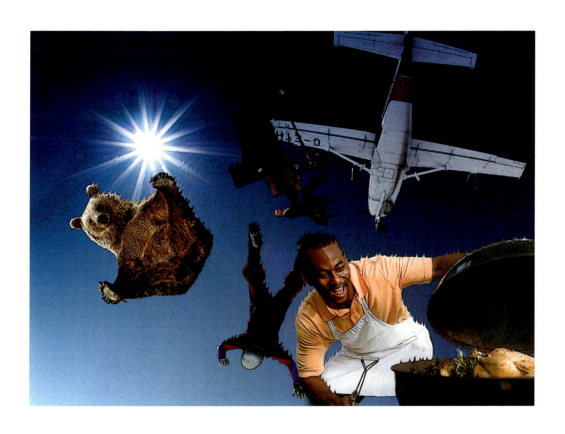

Z62.891

Sibling rivalry

Sarah Bottjen – Acrylic and nailpolish on canvas 11" x 14"
Sarah is currently an Epic project manager on the emergency department team. In her free time, she like to paint with acrylics on found objects. Her largest works are showcased on Epic's campus, where 8 walls exhibit her cave art. She's a French, Chinese and Arabic language fanatic, with a potential interest in emergency medicine in the future.

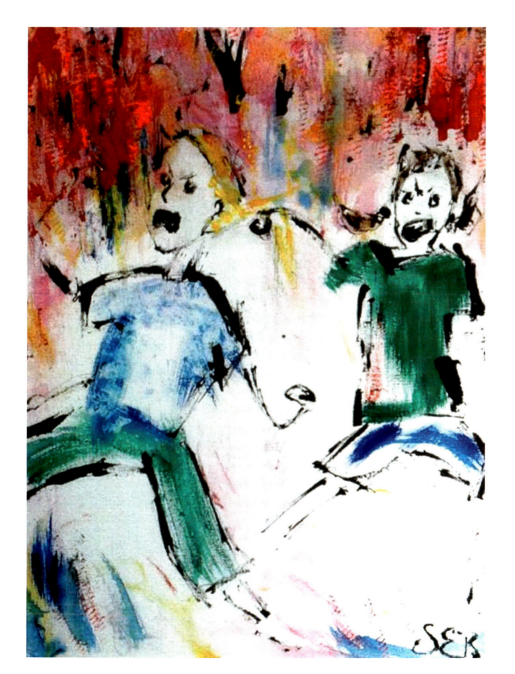

Z63.1

Problems in relationship with in-laws

James Lloyd – Digital
James is the co-founder of 100health and is a wizard with EMR integration. He worked at Epic for six years in various roles including technical services, EDI, and software development. Needless to say, he's a productivity mastermind. In fact, he outsourced his art for this book.

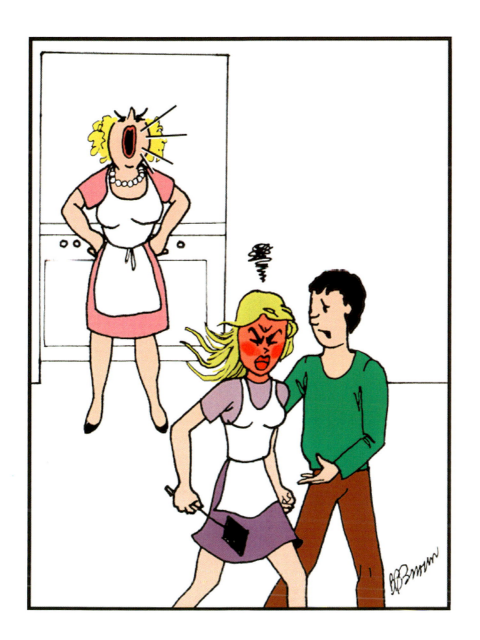

Z73.1

Type A behavior pattern

Erika Samlowski – Digital Media
Erika is a 2nd year medical student at the Medical College of Wisconsin. She is interested in pursuing a career in Reconstructive Surgery.

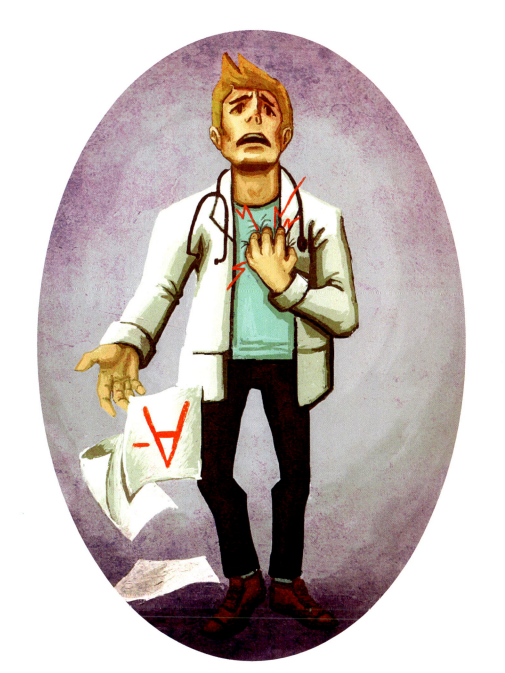

Z73.4

Inadequate social skills, not elsewhere classified

Erika Samlowski – Digital Pencil
Erika is a 2nd year medical student at the Medical College of Wisconsin. She is interested in pursuing a career in Reconstructive Surgery.

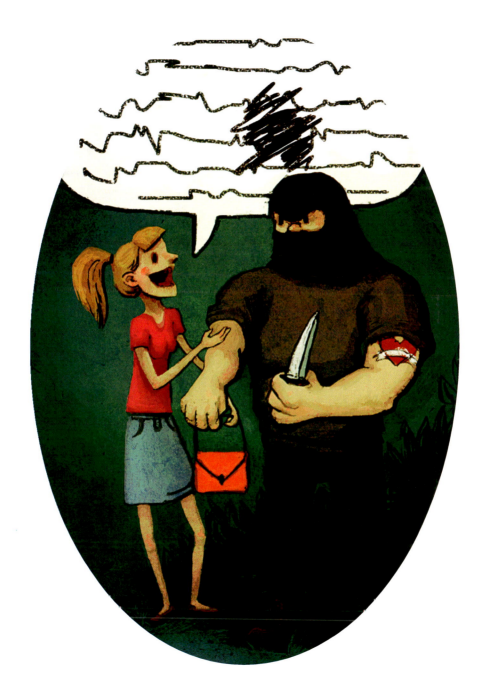

Z89.419

Acquired absence of unspecified great toe

Alex Connelly – Pen, Colored Pencil on Paper 10"x8"
Alex is an artist from Madison, WI. His focus is in digital and analog/experimental photography as well as painting and mixed media.

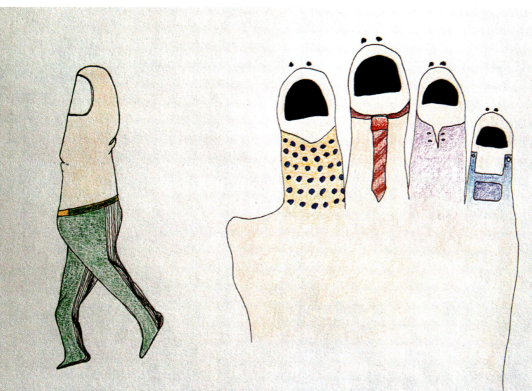

After years of toe-tal bliss, Mr. Hallux put on his best pants and left to discover the world.

Copyright © 2014 by ICD-10 Illustrated LLC
First Edition

Third Print, February 2014

icd10illustrated.com
100 State Street Floor 4
Madison, WI 53703

Special thanks to all of the artists for their brilliance, and to the Madison startup community who never fails to collaborate, engage, and inspire.

ICD-10 Illustrated LLC is a 100 health company.